Incredible Dash Diet Breakfast Recipes for Beginners

Boost Your Metabolism and Start Your Day with Incredibly Fast Recipes

Maya Wilson

Table of contents

Mouthwatering Chicken Porridge

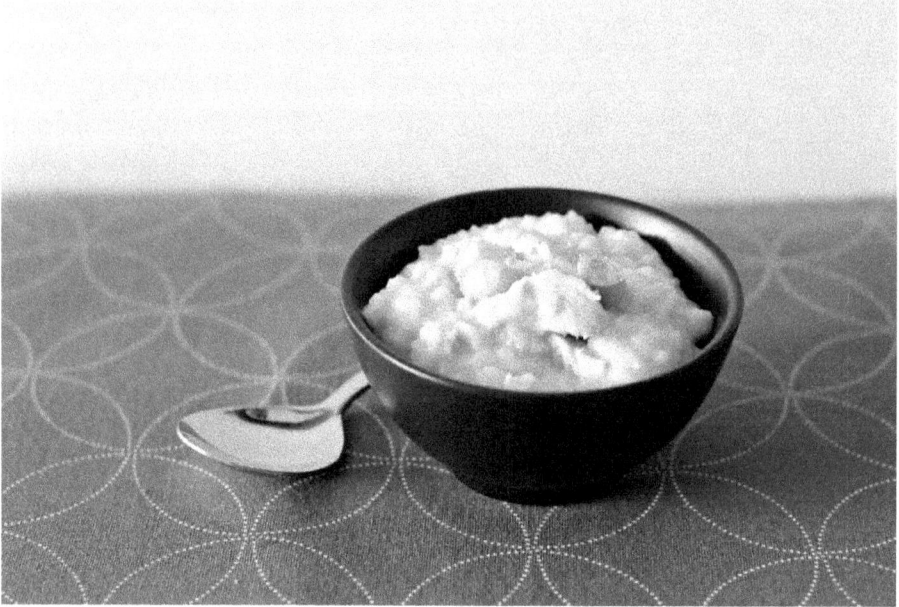

Serving: 4

Prep Time: 1 hour

Cook Time: 10-20 minutes

Ingredients:

- 1 cup jasmine rice

- 1 pound steamed/cooked chicken legs

- 5 cups chicken broth

- 4 cups water

- 1 ½ cups fresh ginger

- Green onions

- Toasted cashew nuts

How To:

1. Place the rice in your fridge and permit it to relax 1 hour before cooking.

2. Take the rice out and add it to your Instant Pot.
3. Pour in chicken stock and water.
4. Lock the lid and cook on PORRIDGE mode, using the default settings and parameters.
5. Release the pressure naturally over 10 minutes.
6. Open the lid.
7. Remove the meat from the chicken legs and add the meat to your soup.
8. Stir overflow Sauté mode.

9. Season with a touch of flavored vinegar and luxuriate in with a garnish of nuts and onion.

Nutrition (Per Serving)

Calories: 206

Fat: 8g

Carbohydrates: 8g

Protein: 23g

Simple Blueberry Oatmeal

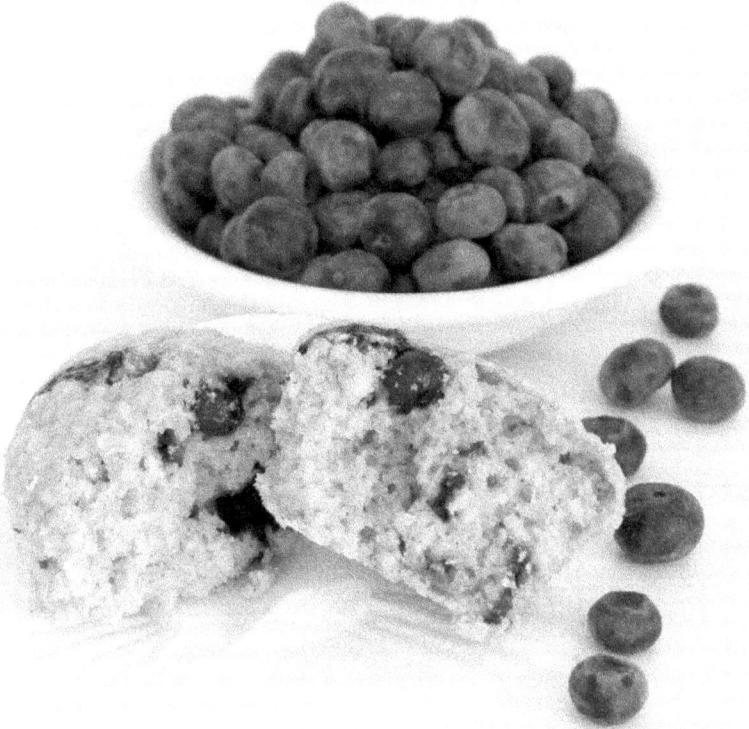

Serving: 4

Prep Time: 10 minutes

Cooking Time: 8 hours

Ingredients:

- 1 cup blueberries

- 1 cup steel-cut oats1 cup coconut milk

- 2 tablespoons agave nectar

- ½ teaspoon vanilla extract Coconut flakes, garnish

How To:

1. Grease Slow Cooker with cooking spray.

2. Add oats, milk, nectar, blueberries, and vanilla.
3. Toss well.
4. Place lid and cook on LOW for 8 hours.
5. Divide between serving bowls and serve.
6. Enjoy!

Nutrition (Per Serving)

Calories: 202

Fat: 6g

Carbohydrates: 12g

Protein: 6g

The Decisive Apple "Porridge"

Serving: 2

Prep Time: 10 minutes

Cook Time: 5 minutes

Ingredients:

- 1 large apple, peeled, cored and grated

- 1 cup unsweetened almond milk

- 1 ½ tablespoons sunflower seeds

- 1/8 cup fresh blueberries

- ¼ teaspoon fresh vanilla bean extract

How To:

1.   Take an outsized pan and add sunflower seeds, vanilla, almond milk, apples, and stir.

2.   Place over medium-low heat.
3.   Cook for five minutes, ensuring to stay the mixture stirring.
4.   Transfer to a serving bowl.
5.   Serve and enjoy!

Nutrition (Per Serving)

Calories: 123

Fat: 1.3g

Carbohydrates:23g

Protein: 4g

The Unique Smoothie Bowl

Serving: 2

Prep Time: 10 minutes

Cook Time: Nil

Ingredients:

- 2 cups baby spinach leaves

- 1 cup coconut almond milk

- ¼ cup low fat cream

- 2 tablespoons flaxseed oil

- 2 tablespoons chia seeds

- 2 tablespoons walnuts, roughly chopped A handful of fresh berries

How To:
1.   Add spinach leaves, coconut almond milk, cream and linseed oil to a blender.

2.   Blitz until smooth.
3.   Pour smoothie into serving bowls.
4.   Sprinkle chia seeds, berries, walnuts on top.

5.   Serve and enjoy!

Nutrition (Per Serving)

Calories: 380

Fat: 36g

Carbohydrates: 12g

Protein: 5g

Cinnamon and Coconut Porridge

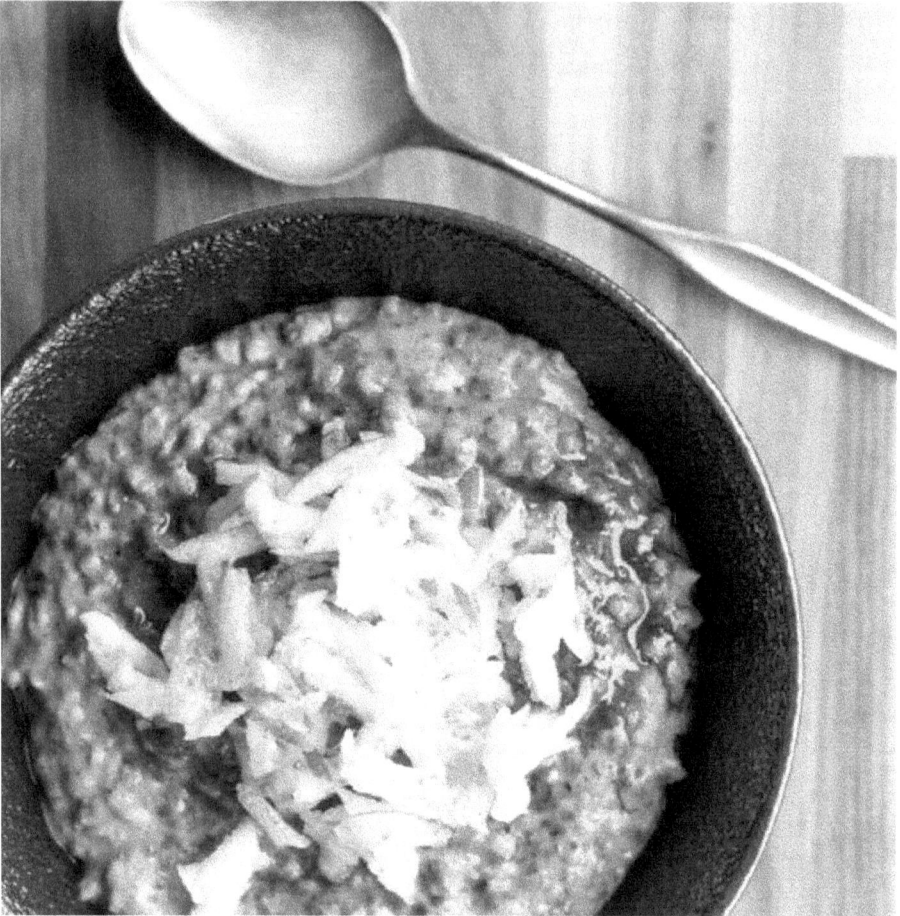

Serving: 4

Prep Time: 5 minutes

Cook Time:5 minutes

Ingredients:

- 2 cups water

- 1 cup coconut cream

- ½ cup unsweetened dried coconut, shredded

- 2 tablespoons flaxseed meal 1 tablespoon almond butter

- 1 ½ teaspoons stevia

- 1 teaspoon cinnamon

- Toppings as blueberries

How To:

1.   Add the listed ingredients to alittle pot, mix well.

2.   Transfer pot to stove and place over medium-low heat.
3.   bring back mix to a slow boil.
4.   Stir well and take away from the warmth .
5.   Divide the combination into equal servings and allow them to sit for 10 minutes.
6.   Top together with your desired toppings and enjoy!

Nutrition (Per Serving)

Calories: 171

Fat: 16g

Carbohydrates: 6g

Protein: 2g

Morning Porridge

Serving: 2

Prep Time: 15 minutes

Cook Time: Nil

Ingredients:

- 2 tablespoons coconut flour

- 2 tablespoons vanilla protein powder

- 3 tablespoons Golden Flaxseed meal

- 1 ½ cups almond milk, unsweetened Powdered erythritol

How To:

1.   Take a bowl and blend in flaxseed meal, protein powder, coconut flour and blend well.

2.   Add mix to the saucepan (place over medium heat).
3.   Add almond milk and stir, let the mixture thicken .
4.   Add your required amount of sweetener and serve.
5.   Enjoy!

Nutrition (Per Serving)

Calories: 259

Fat: 13g

Carbohydrates: 5g

Protein: 16g

Vanilla Sweet Potato Porridge

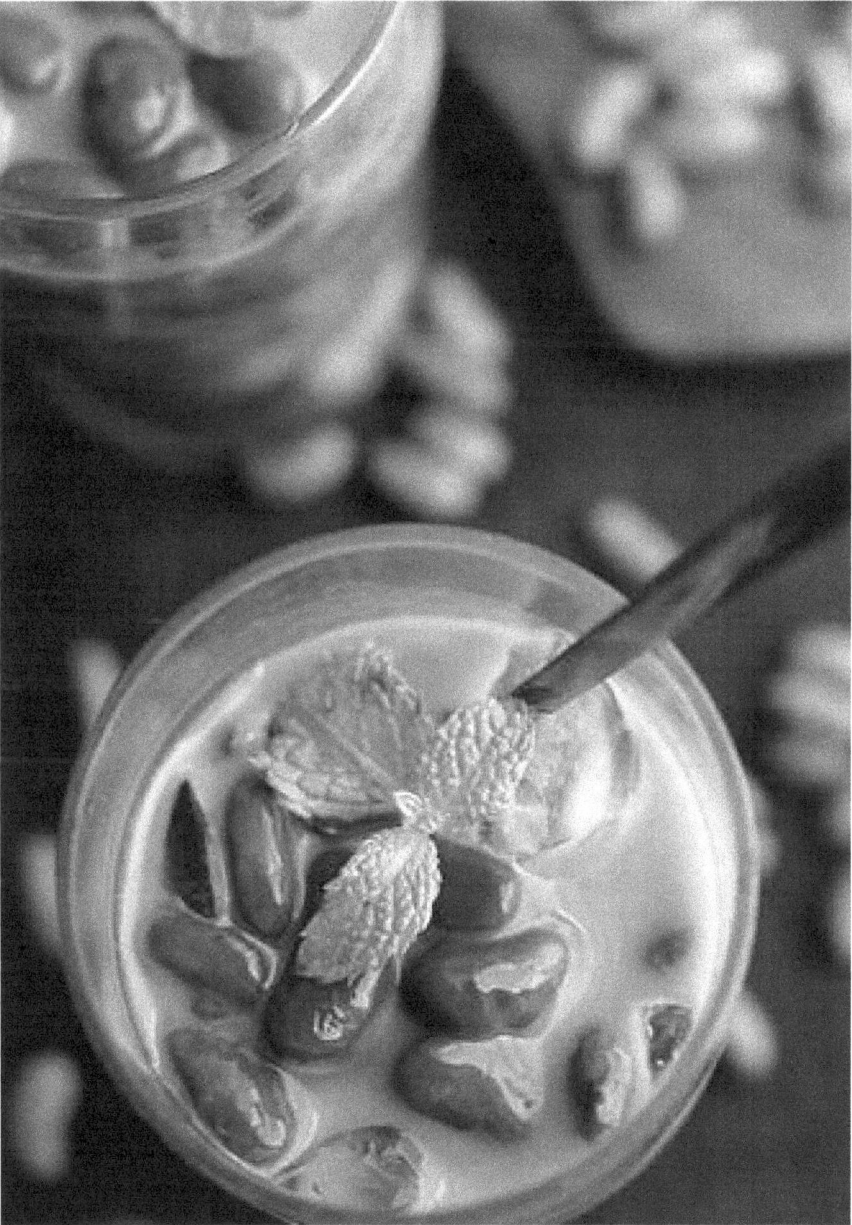

Serving: 5

Prep Time: 10 minutes

Cook Time: 8 hours

Ingredients:

- 6 sweet potatoes, peeled and cut into 1-inch cubes

- 1 ½ cups light coconut milk

- 1 teaspoon ground cinnamon

- 1 teaspoon ground cardamom

- 1 teaspoon pure vanilla extract

- 1 cup raisins Pinch of salt

How To:
1.   Add sweet potatoes coconut milk, vanilla, cardamom, cinnamon to your Slow Cooker.

2.   Close lid and cook on LOW for 8 hours.
3.   Open the lid and mash the entire mixture using potato masher to mash the sweet potatoes, stir well.
4.   Stir in raisins, salt and serve.

5.   Serve and enjoy!

Nutrition (Per Serving)

Calories: 317

Fat: 4g

Carbohydrates: 71g

Protein: 4g

A Nice German Oatmeal

Serving: 3

Prep Time: 10 minutes

Cook Time: 8 hours

Ingredients:

- 1 cup steel-cut oats

- 3 cups water

- 6 ounces coconut milk

- 2 tablespoons cocoa powder

- 1 tablespoon brown sugar

- 1 tablespoon coconut, shredded

How to

1.   Grease the Slow Cooker well.

2.   Add the listed ingredients to your Cooker and stir.

3.   Place lid and cook on LOW for 8 hours.
4.   Divide amongst serving bowls and enjoy!

Nutrition (Per Serving)

Calories: 200

Fat: 4g

Carbohydrates: 11g

Protein: 5g

Very Nutty Banana Oatmeal

Serving: 4

Prep Time: 15 minutes

Cook Time: 7-9 hours

Ingredients:

- 1 cup steel-cut oats

- 1 ripe banana, mashed

- 2 cups unsweetened almond milk

- 1 cup water

- 1 ½ tablespoons honey

- ½ teaspoon vanilla extract

- ¼ cup almonds, chopped

- 1 teaspoon ground cinnamon

- ¼ teaspoon ground nutmeg

How To:

1. Grease the Slow Cooker well.

2. Add the listed ingredients to your Slow Cooker and stir.

3. Cover with lid and cook on LOW for 7-9 hours.
4. Serve and enjoy!

Nutrition (Per Serving)

Calories: 230

Fat: 7g

Carbohydrates: 40g

Protein: 5g

Cool Coconut Flatbread

Serving: 4

Prep Time: 15 minutes

Cooking Time: 10 minutes

Ingredients:

- 1 ½ tablespoons coconut flour

- ¼ teaspoon baking powder

- 1/8 teaspoon sunflower seeds

- 1 tablespoon coconut oil, melted

- 1 whole egg

How To:

1.   Preheat your oven to 350 degrees F.

2.   Add coconut flour, leaven , sunflower seeds.
3.   Add copra oil , eggs and stir well until mixed.
4.   Leave the batter for several minutes.
5.   Pour half the batter onto the baking pan.
6.   Spread it to make a circle, repeat with remaining batter.
7.   Bake within the oven for 10 minutes.
8.   Once you get a golden-brown texture, let it cool and serve.
9.   Enjoy!

Nutrition (Per Serving)

Total Carbs: 9 (%)

Fiber: 3g

Protein: 8g (%)

Fat: 20g (%)

Perfect Homemade Pickled Ginger Gari

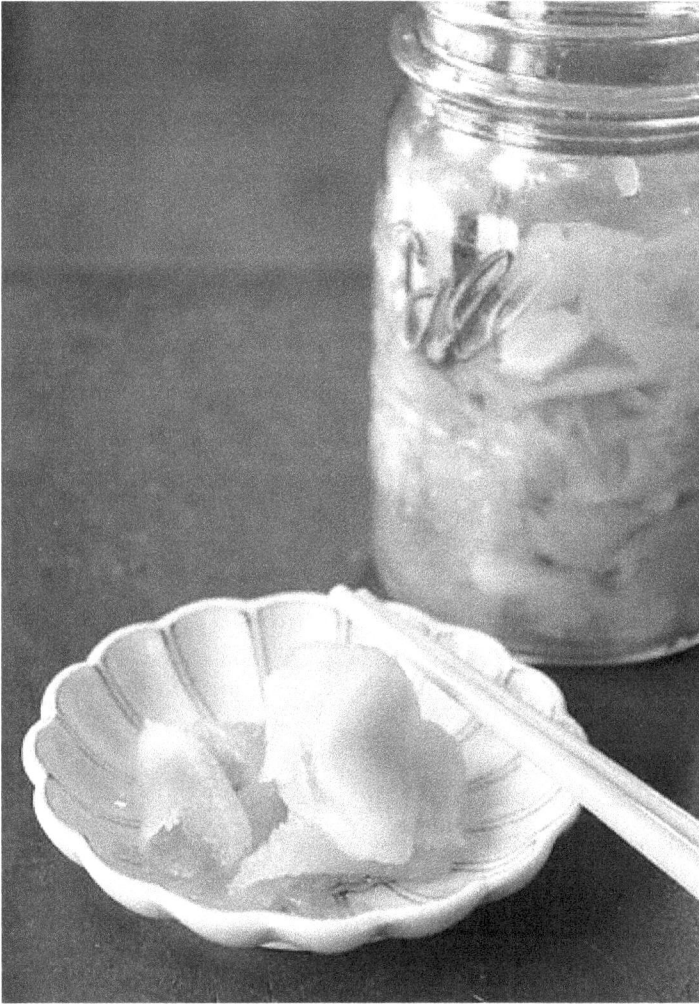

Serving: 8

Prep Time: 40 minute

Cook Time: 5 minutes

Ingredients:

- About 8 ounces of fresh ginger root, completely peeled

- 1 teaspoon and extra ½ teaspoon of fine sunflower seeds

- 1 cup vinegar, rice

- 1/3 cup sugar, white

How To:

1.   Cut your ginger into small-sized chunks and transfer them to a bowl.

2.   Season with sunflower seeds and stir, let the mixture sit for a minimum of half-hour .
3.   Take a saucepan and add sugar and vinegar, heat it up, bring the mixture to a boil and keep boiling until the sugar has completely dissolved.
4.   Pour the liquid over your ginger pieces.
5.   Let it cool and wait until the water changes color.
6.   Enjoy!
7.   Alternatively, store in jars and use as required .

Nutrition (Per Serving)

Calories: 14

Fat: 0.1g

Carbohydrates: 3g

Protein: 0.1g

Avocado and Blueberry Medley

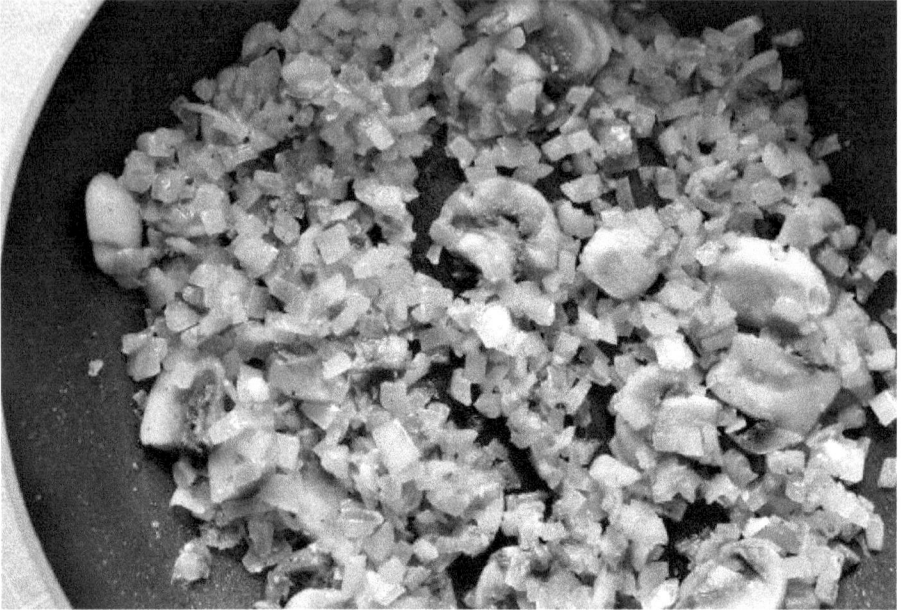

Serving: 4

Prep Time: 5 minutes

Cook Time: Nil

Ingredients:

- 1 frozen banana

- 2 avocados, quartered

- 2 cups berries

- Maple syrup as needed

How To:

1.   Take your blender and add all ingredients except syrup.

2.   Add drinking water and blend.
3.   Garnish with syrup and pour in smoothie glasses.
4.   Enjoy!

Nutrition (Per Serving)

Calories: 250

Fat: 13g

Carbohydrates: 40g

Protein 4g

Healthy Zucchini Stir Fry

Serving: 4

Prep Time: 10 minutes

Cook Time: 10 minutes

Ingredients:

- 2 heaped tablespoons olive oil

- 1 medium-sized onion, sliced thinly

- 2 medium-sized zucchini, cut up into thin sized strips

- 2 heaped tablespoons teriyaki flavored sauce, low sodium

1 tablespoon coconut aminos

1 tablespoon sesame seed, toasted Ground pepper (black) as much as needed
How To:

1. Take a skillet and place it over medium level heat.

2. Add onions, and stir-cook for five minutes.
3. Add your zucchini and stir-cook for 1 minute more.
4. Gently add the sauces alongside the sesame seeds.
5. Cook for five minutes more until the zucchini are soft.
6. Finally, add the pepper and enjoy!

Nutrition (Per Serving)

Calories: 110

Fat: 9g

Carbohydrates: 8g

Protein: 3g

Herbed Parmesan Walnuts

Serving: 4

Prep Time: 5 minutes

Cook Time: 30 minutes

Ingredients:

- ½ cup kite ricotta/cashew cheese

- ½ teaspoon Italian herb seasoning and garlic sunflower seeds

- 1 teaspoon parsley flakes

- 2 cups walnuts

1 egg white

How To:

1.   Preheat your oven to 250 degrees F.

2.   Take a bowl and add all ingredients except the albumen and walnuts.
3.   Whisk within the albumen , stir in halved walnuts and blend well.

4.   Transfer the mixture to a greased baking sheet and bake for half-hour .

5.   Serve and enjoy!

Nutrition (Per Serving)

Calories: 220

Fat: 21g

Carbohydrates: 4g

Protein 8g

Amazing Scrambled Turkey Eggs

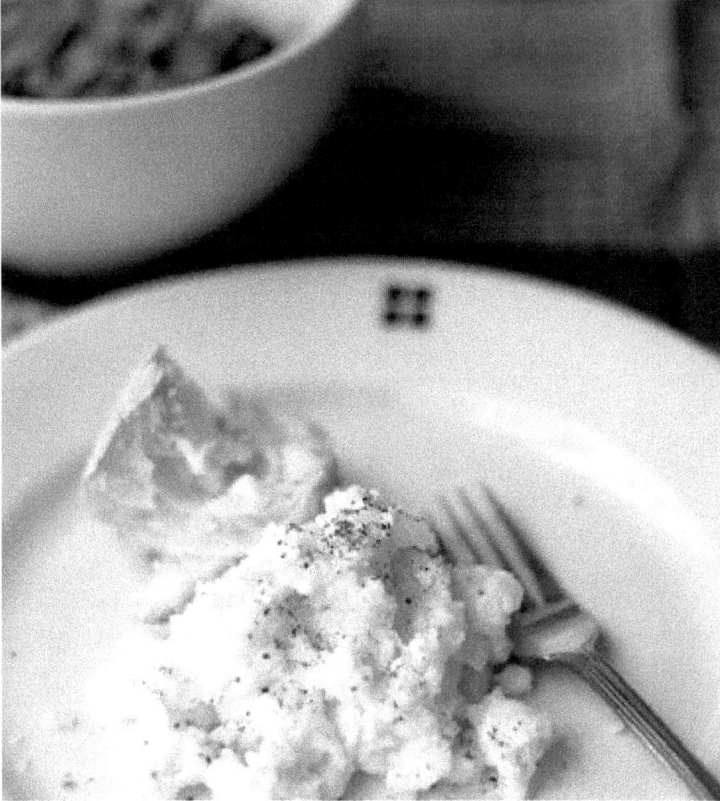

Serving: 2

Prep Time: 15 minutes

Cook Time: 15 minutes

Ingredients:

- 1 tablespoon coconut oil

- 1 medium red bell pepper, diced

- ½ medium yellow onion, diced

- ¼ teaspoon hot pepper sauce

- 3 large free-range eggs

- ¼ teaspoon black pepper, freshly ground

- ¼ teaspoon salt

How To:

1.   Set a pan to medium-high heat, add copra oil , let it heat up.

2.   Add onions and sauté.
3.   Add turkey and red pepper .

4.   Cook until the turkey is cooked.

5.   Take a bowl and beat eggs, stir in salt and pepper.
6.   Pour eggs within the pan with turkey and gently cook and scramble eggs.
7.   Top with sauce and enjoy!

Nutrition (Per Serving)

Calories: 435

Fat: 30g

Carbohydrates: 34g

Protein: 16g

Egg and Bacon Cups

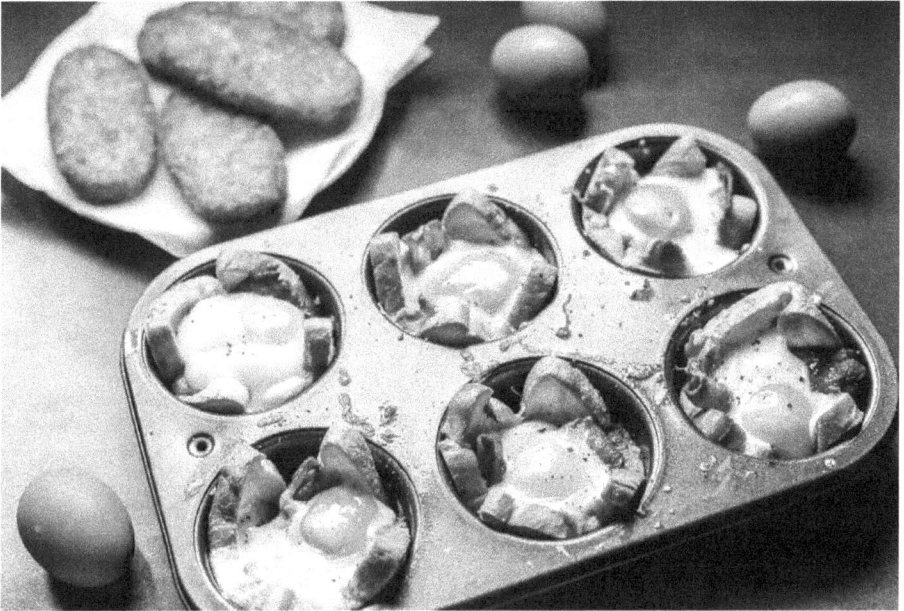

Serving: 6

Prep Time: 10 minutes

Cook Time: 15 minutes

Ingredients:

- 2 bacon strips

- 2 large eggs

- A handful of fresh spinach

- ¼ cup cheese

- Salt and pepper to taste

How To:

1. Preheat your oven to 400 degrees F.

2. Fry bacon during a skillet over medium heat, drain the oil and keep them on the side.
3. Take muffin tin and grease with oil.
4. Line with a slice of bacon, depress the bacon well, ensuring that the ends are protruding (to be used as handles).
5. Take a bowl and beat eggs.
6. Drain and pat the spinach dry.
7. Add the spinach to the eggs.
8. Add 1 / 4 of the mixture in each of your muffin tins.

9. Sprinkle cheese and season.

10. Bake for quarter-hour .
11. Enjoy!

Nutrition (Per Serving)

Calories: 101

Fat: 7g

Carbohydrates: 2g

Protein: 8g

Fiber: 1g

Net Carbs: 1g

Pepperoni Omelet

Serving: 2

Prep Time: 5 minutes

Cook Time: 20 minutes

Ingredients:

- 3 eggs

- 7 pepperoni slices

- 1 teaspoon coconut cream

- Salt and freshly ground black pepper, to taste
- 1 tablespoons butter

How To:

1.	Take a bowl and whisk eggs with all the remaining ingredients in it.

2.	Then take a skillet and warmth the butter.
3.	Pour ¼ of the egg mixture into your skillet.
4.	After that, cook for two minutes per side.
5.	Repeat to use the whole batter.
6.	Serve warm and enjoy!

Nutrition (Per Serving)

Calories: 141

Fat: 11.5g

Carbohydrates: 0.6g

Protein: 8.9g

Cinnamon Baked Apple Chips

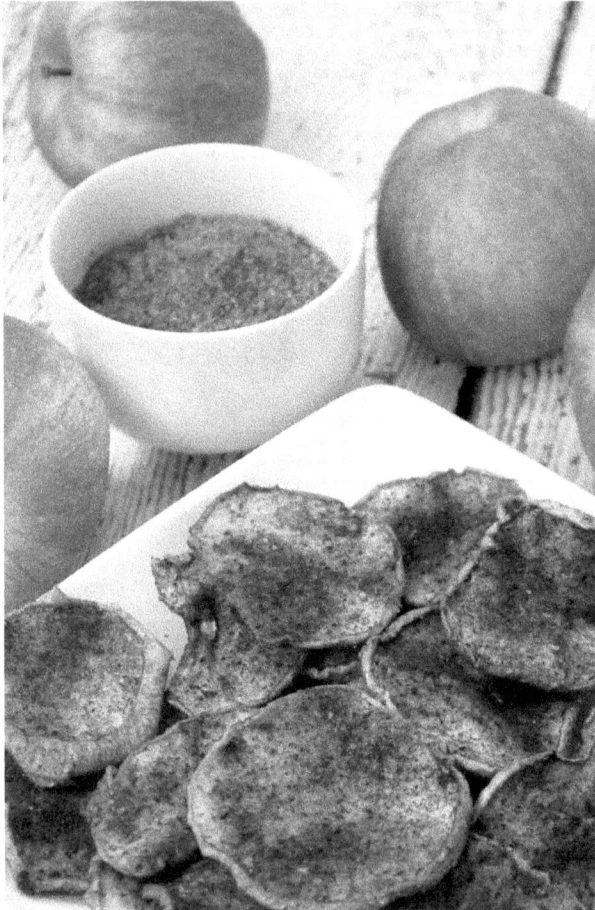

Serving: 2

Prep Time: 5 minutes

Cook Time: 2 hours

Ingredients:

- 1 teaspoon cinnamon

- 1-2 apples

How To:

1.   Preheat your oven to 200 degrees F.

2.   Take a pointy knife and slice apples into thin slices.
3.   Discard seeds.
4.   Line a baking sheet with parchment paper and arrange apples thereon .
5.   Confirm they are doing not overlap.
6.   Once done, sprinkle cinnamon over apples.
7.   Bake within the oven for 1 hour.
8.   Flip and bake for an hour more until not moist.
9.   Serve and enjoy!

Nutrition (Per Serving)

Calories: 147

Fat: 0g

Carbohydrates: 39g

Protein: 1g

Herb and Avocado Omelet

Serving: 2

Prep Time: 2 minutes

Cook Time: 10 minutes

Ingredients:

- 3 large free-range eggs

- ½ medium avocado, sliced

- ½ cup almonds, sliced

- Salt and pepper as needed

How To:

1.   Take a non-stick skillet and place it over medium-high heat.

2.   Take a bowl and add eggs, beat the eggs.
3.   Pour into the skillet and cook for 1 minute.
4.   Reduce heat to low and cook for 4 minutes.
5.   Top the omelet with almonds and avocado.
6.   Sprinkle salt and pepper and serve.
7.   Enjoy!

Nutrition (Per Serving)

Calories: 193

Fat: 15g

Carbohydrates: 5g

Protein: 10g

Classic Apple and Cinnamon Oatmeal

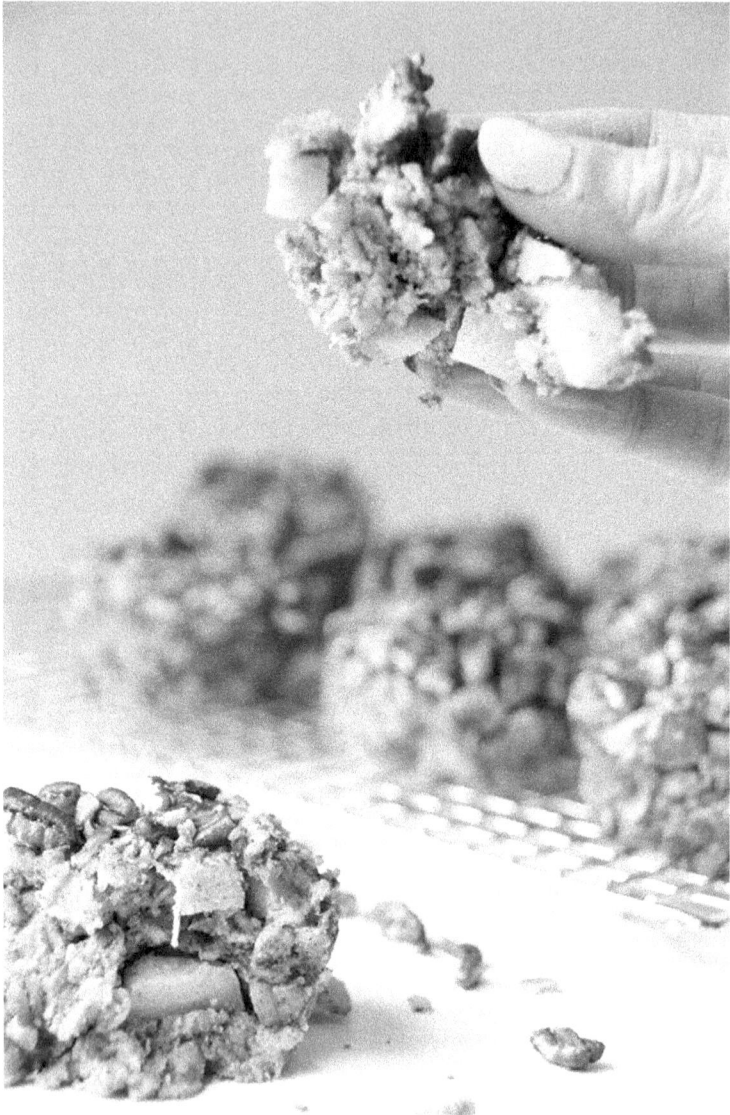

Serving: 4

Prep Time: 15 minutes

Cook Time: 7-9 hours

Ingredients:

- 1 apple, cored, peeled and diced

- 1 cup steel-cut oats

- 2 ½ cups unsweetened vanilla almond milk

- 2 tablespoons honey

- ½ teaspoon vanilla extract

- 1 teaspoon ground cinnamon

How To:

1.   Grease the Slow Cooker well.

2.   Add the listed ingredients to your Slow Cooker and stir.
3.   Cover with lid and cook on LOW for 7-9 hours.
4.   Serve and enjoy!

Nutrition (Per Serving)

Calories: 126

Fat: 3g

Carbohydrates: 25g

Protein: 3g

Carrot and Zucchini Oatmeal

Serving: 3

Prep Time: 10 minutes

Cook Time: 8 hours

Ingredients:

- ½ cup steel cut oats

- 1 cup coconut milk

- 1 carrot, grated

- ¼ zucchini, grated

- Pinch of nutmeg

- ½ teaspoon cinnamon powder

- 2 tablespoons brown sugar

- ¼ cup pecans, chopped

How To:

1.   Grease the Slow Cooker well.

2.   Add oats, zucchini, milk, carrot, nutmeg, cloves, sugar, cinnamon and stir well.
3.   Place lid and cook on LOW for 8 hours.

4. Divide amongst serving bowls and enjoy!

Nutrition (Per Serving)

Calories: 200

Fat: 4g

Carbohydrates: 11g

Protein: 5g

Blueberry and Walnut "Steel" Oatmeal

Serving: 8

Prep Time: 5 minutes

Cook Time: 7-8 hours

Ingredients:

- 2 cups steel-cut oats

- 6 cups water

- 2 cups low-fat milk

- 2 cups fresh blueberries

- 1 ripe banana, mashed

- 1 teaspoon vanilla extract

- 2 teaspoons ground cinnamon

- 2 tablespoons brown sugar

- Pinch of salt

- ½ cup walnuts, chopped

How To:

1.   Grease the within of your Slow Cooker.

2.   Add oats, milk, water, blueberries, banana, vanilla, sugar , cinnamon and salt to your Slow Cooker.
3.   Stir.
4.   Place lid and cook on LOW for 7-8 hours.
5.   Serve warm with a garnish of chopped walnuts.
6.   Enjoy!

Nutrition (Per Serving)

Calories: 372

Fat: 14g

Carbohydrates: 56g

Protein: 8g

Shrimp and Egg Medley

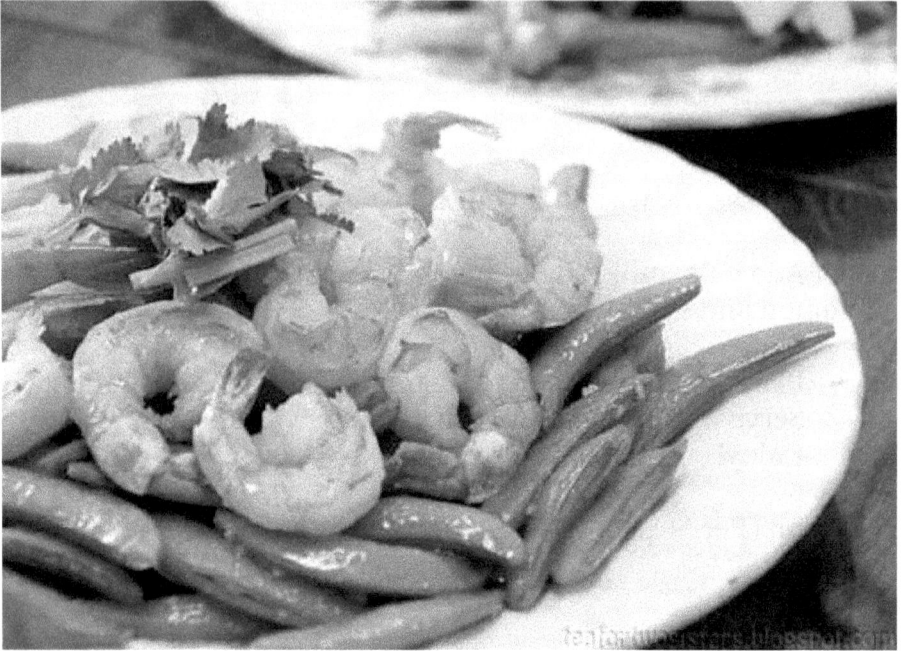

Serving: 4

Prep Time: 15 minutes

Cook Time: nil

Ingredients:

- 4 hardboiled eggs, peeled and chopped

- 1-pound cooked shrimp, peeled and de-veined, chopped

- 1 sprig fresh dill, chopped

- ¼ cup mayonnaise

- 1 teaspoon Dijon mustard

- 4 fresh lettuce leaves

How To:

1.   Take an outsized serving bowl and add the listed ingredients (except lettuce.)

2.   Stir well.
3.   Serve over bet of lettuce leaves.
4.   Enjoy!

Nutrition (Per Serving)

Calories: 292

Fat: 17g

Carbohydrates: 1.6g

Protein: 30g

Crispy Walnut Crumbles

Serving: 10

Prep Time: 10 minutes

Cook Time: 8 minutes

Ingredients:

- 6 ounces kite ricotta/cashew cheese, grated

- 2 tablespoons walnuts, chopped

- 1 tablespoon almond butter

- ½ tablespoon fresh thyme chopped

How To:

1.   Preheat your oven to 350 degrees F.

2.   Take two large rimmed baking sheets and line with parchment.

3.   Add cheese, almond butter to a kitchen appliance and blend.

4.   Add walnuts to the combination and pulse.
5.   Take a tablespoon and scoop mix onto a baking sheet.
6.   Top them with chopped thymes.
7.   Bake for 8 minutes, transfer to a cooling rack.

8.   Let it cool for half-hour .
9.   Serve and enjoy!

Nutrition (Per Serving)

Calories: 80

Fat: 3g

Carbohydrates: 7g

Protein: 7g

Cheesy Zucchini Omelette

Serving: 3

Prep Time: 10 minutes

Cook Time: 20 minutes

Ingredients:

- 4 large eggs

- 2-3 medium zucchinis

- 1-2 garlic cloves, crushed

- 4 tablespoons grated cheese Season as needed

How To:

1.   Take a bowl and add grated zucchinis, confirm to peel them because the skin is bitter.

2.   Take a bowl and break within the eggs, crushed garlic and cheese.

3.   Pour the mixture during a hot frypan with a touch little bit of oil and place it over medium heat, keep a lid on.
4.   Once the egg is cooked nicely, and therefore the bottom is crispy and golden, serve and luxuriate in with a garnish of chopped parsley.
5.   Enjoy!

Nutrition (Per Serving)

Calories: 289

Fat: 20g

Carbohydrates: 7g

Protein: 21g

Old Fashioned Breakfast Oatmeal

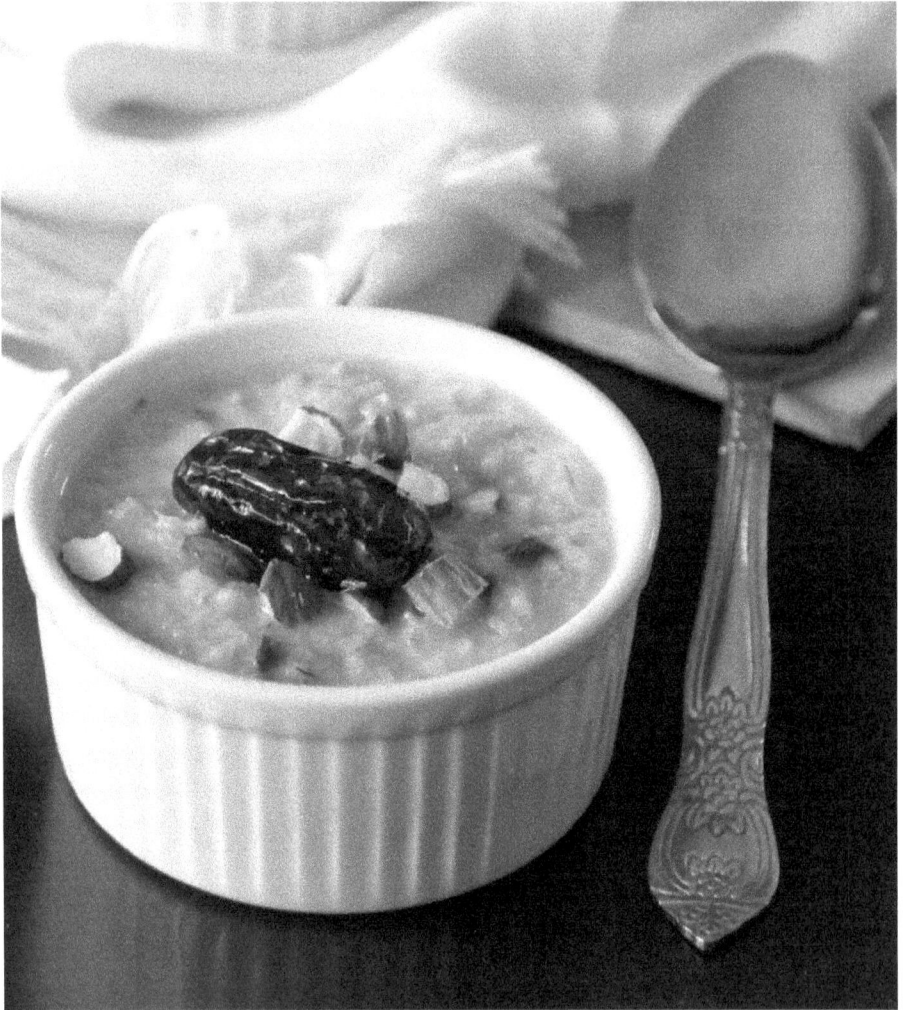

Serving: 4

Prep Time: 10 minutes

Cook Time: 5 minutes

Ingredients:

- 2 ½ cups water

- 1 cup old fashioned oats

- 1 cup apple, peeled, cored and chopped

- 3 tablespoons low-fat butter

- 2 tablespoons palm sugar

- ½ teaspoon cinnamon powder

How To:

1. Add water, oats, apple, butter, cinnamon, and sugar to a moment

Pot.

2. Toss well and lock the lid.

3. Cook on high for five minutes.
4. Release the pressure naturally over 10 minutes.
5. Stir oats and divide into bowls.
6. Enjoy!

Nutrition (Per Serving)

Calories: 191

Fat: 2g

Carbohydrates: 9g

Protein: 5g

Healthy Peach Oatmeal

Serving: 8

Prep Time: 10 minutes

Cook Time: 10 minutes

Ingredients:

4 cups old fashioned rolled oats

- 3 ½ cups low-fat milk

- 3 ½ cups water

- 1 teaspoon cinnamon powder

- 1/3 cup palm sugar

- 4 peaches, chopped

How To:

1.   Add oats, milk, cinnamon, water, sugar, and peaches to your Instant Pot.

2.   Toss well.
3.   Lock the lid and cook for 10 minutes on high .
4.   Release the pressure naturally over 10 minutes .
5.   Divide the combination in bowls and serve!

Nutrition (Per Serving)

Calories: 192

Fat: 3g

Carbohydrates: 12g

Protein: 4g

Fancy Banana Oatmeal

Serving: 4

Prep Time: 10 minutes

Cook Time: 10 minutes

Ingredients:

- 2 cups water

- 1 cup steel-cut oats

- 1 cup almond milk

- ¼ cup walnuts, chopped

- 2 tablespoons flaxseeds, ground

- 2 tablespoons chia seeds

- 2 bananas, peeled and mashed

- 1 teaspoon vanilla extract

- 1 teaspoon cinnamon powder

How To:

1.   Add water, oats, almond milk, flaxseed, walnuts, chia seeds, vanilla, bananas, cinnamon to your Instant Pot and provides it a pleasant toss.
2.   Lock the lid and cook on high for 10 minutes.
3.   Release the pressure naturally and open the lid.
4.   Divide the combination amongst bowls and serve.
5.   Enjoy!

Nutrition (Per Serving)

Calories: 200

Fat: 4g

Carbohydrates: 11g

Protein: 4g

Traditional Frittata

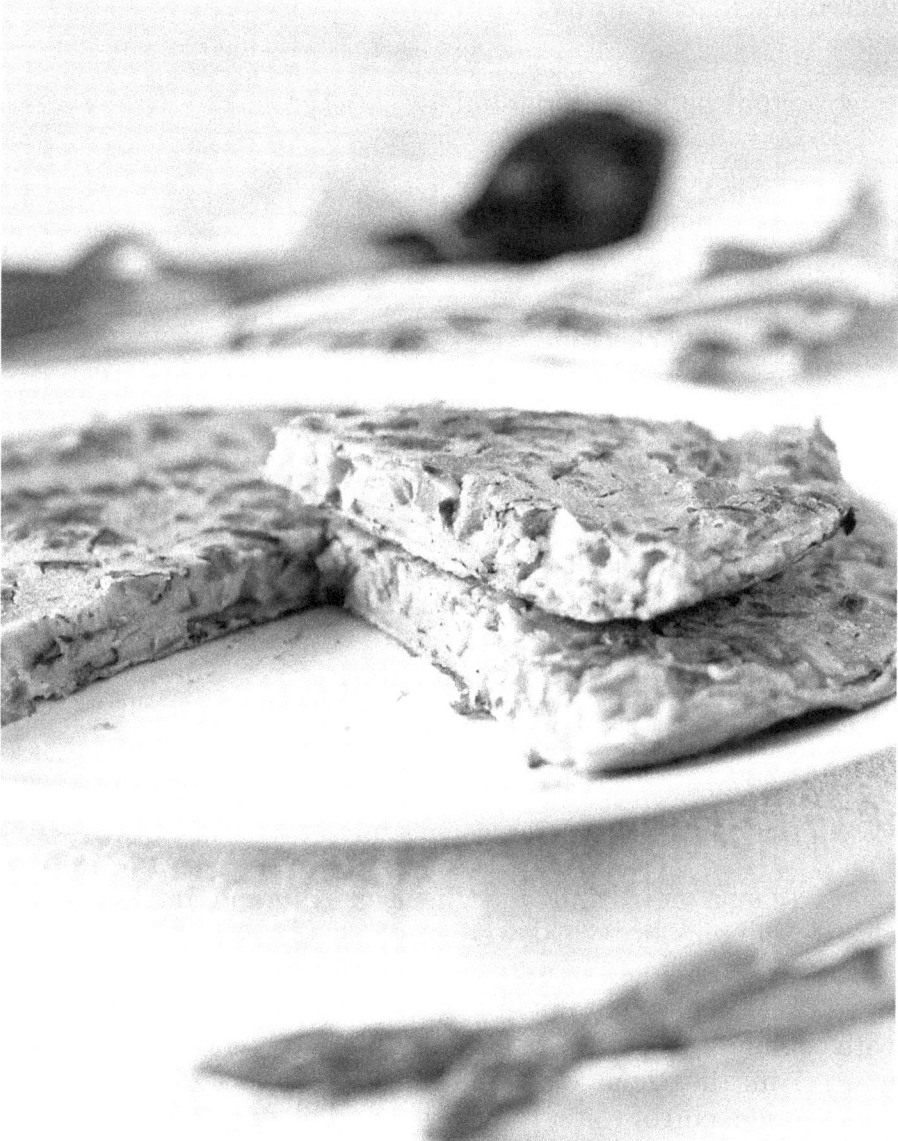

Serving: 6

Prep Time: 10 minutes

Cook Time: 5 minutes

Ingredients:

- 2 tablespoons almond milk

- Just a pinch pepper

- 6 eggs, cracked and whisked

- 2 tablespoons parsley, chopped

- 1 tablespoon low-fat cheese, shredded

- 1 cup of water

How To:

1.   Take a bowl and add the eggs, almond milk, pepper, cheese, and parsley. Whisk well.

2.   Take a pan that might slot in your Instant Pot and grease with cooking spray.
3.   Pour the egg mix into the pan.
4.   Add a cup of water to your pot and place a steamer basket.
5.   Add the pan within the basket.
6.   Lock the lid and cook on high for five minutes.
7.   Release the pressure naturally over 10 minutes.
8.   Remove the lid and divide the frittata amongst serving plates.

9.   Enjoy!

Nutrition (Per Serving)

Calories: 200

Fat: 4g

Carbohydrates: 17g

Protein: 6g

Pepperoni Omelet

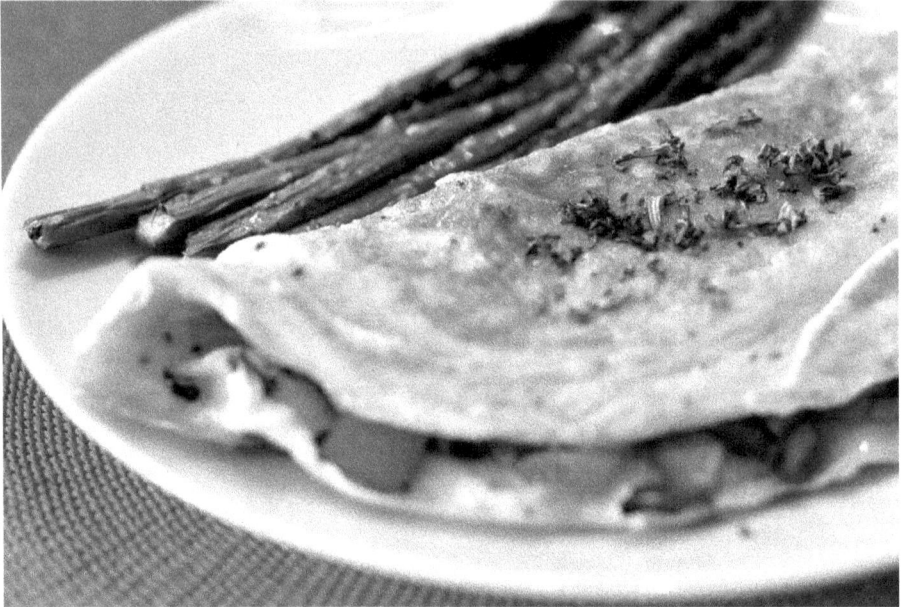

Serving: 2

Prep Time: 5 minutes

Cook Time: 20 minutes

Ingredients:

- 3 eggs

- 7 pepperoni slices

- 1 teaspoon coconut cream

- Salt and freshly ground black pepper, to taste

- 1 tablespoon butter

How To:

1.   Take a bowl and whisk eggs with all the remaining ingredients in it.

2.   Then take a skillet and warmth butter.
3.   Pour quarter of the egg mixture into your skillet.
4.   After that, cook for two minutes per side.
5.   Repeat to use the whole batter.
6.   Serve warm and enjoy!

Nutrition (Per Serving)

Calories: 141

Fat: 11.5g

Carbohydrates: 0.6g

Protein: 8.9g

Eggy Tomato Scramble

Serving: 2

Prep Time: 10 minutes

Cook Time: 5 minutes

Ingredients:

- 2 whole eggs

- ½ cup fresh basil, chopped

- 2 tablespoons olive oil

- ½ teaspoon red pepper flakes, crushed

- 1 cup grape tomatoes, chopped

- Salt and pepper to taste

How To:

1.   Take a bowl and whisk in eggs, salt, pepper, red pepper flakes and blend well.

2.   Add tomatoes, basil, and mix.
3.   Take a skillet and place over medium-high heat.

4.   Add the egg mixture and cook for five minutes until cooked and scrambled.

5.   Enjoy!

Nutrition (Per Serving)

Calories: 130

Fat: 10g

Carbohydrates: 8g

Protein: 1.8g

Breakfast Fruit Pizzas

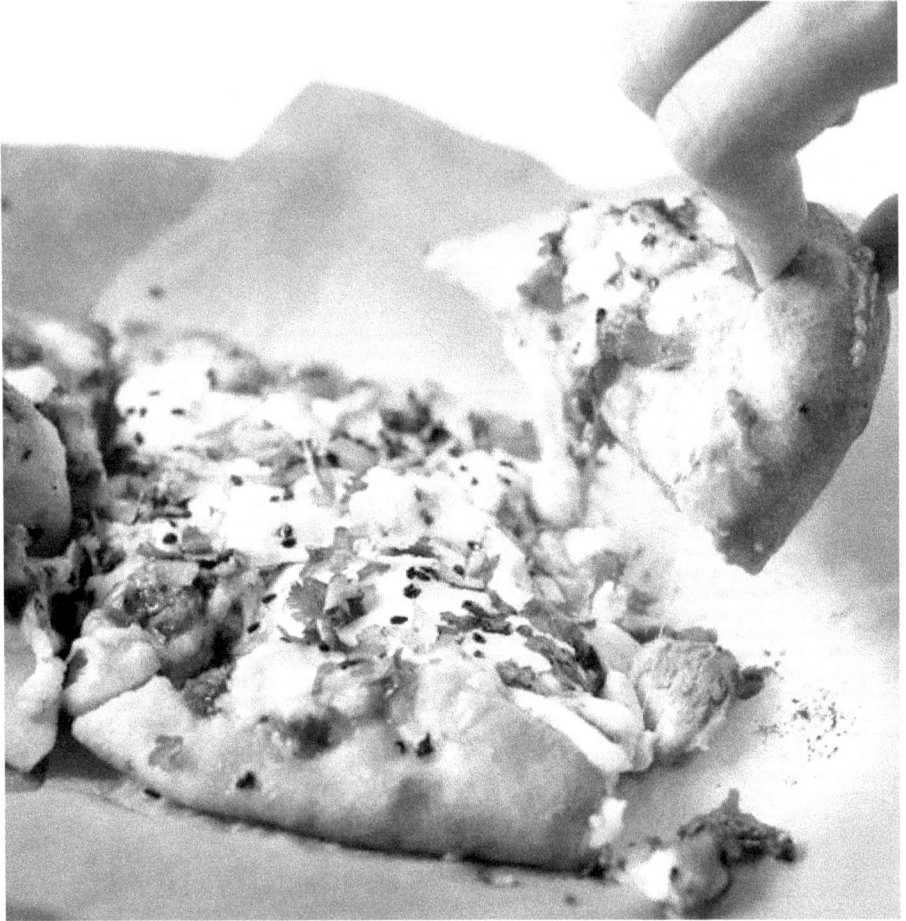

Ingredients

- Two whole-wheat pita flatbreads

- 7 ounces Arla Original Cream Cheese

- 1-2 teaspoons honey

- 1/2 teaspoon pure vanilla extract

- Three kiwi skin removed and sliced

- 1/2 cup sliced strawberries

- 1/2 cup blackberries

- 1/4 cup blueberries

- Two raspberries for the center

Instructions

1.   Preheat the oven to broil. Put the entire wheat pita flatbreads within the oven. Broil for 1 minute and switch over. Broilfor one minute more. you'll also toast the entire pita bread during a kitchen appliance . Set the dough aside to chill.

2.   Take a bowl and blend the cheese , honey, and vanilla. Spread the cheese on the pita bread.
3.   Decorate the fruit on top of the cheese . dig slices and serve immediately.
4.   Note-you can use your favorite fruit. Bananas, peaches, pineapple, oranges, nectarines would even be good!

Peanut Butter Overnight Oats

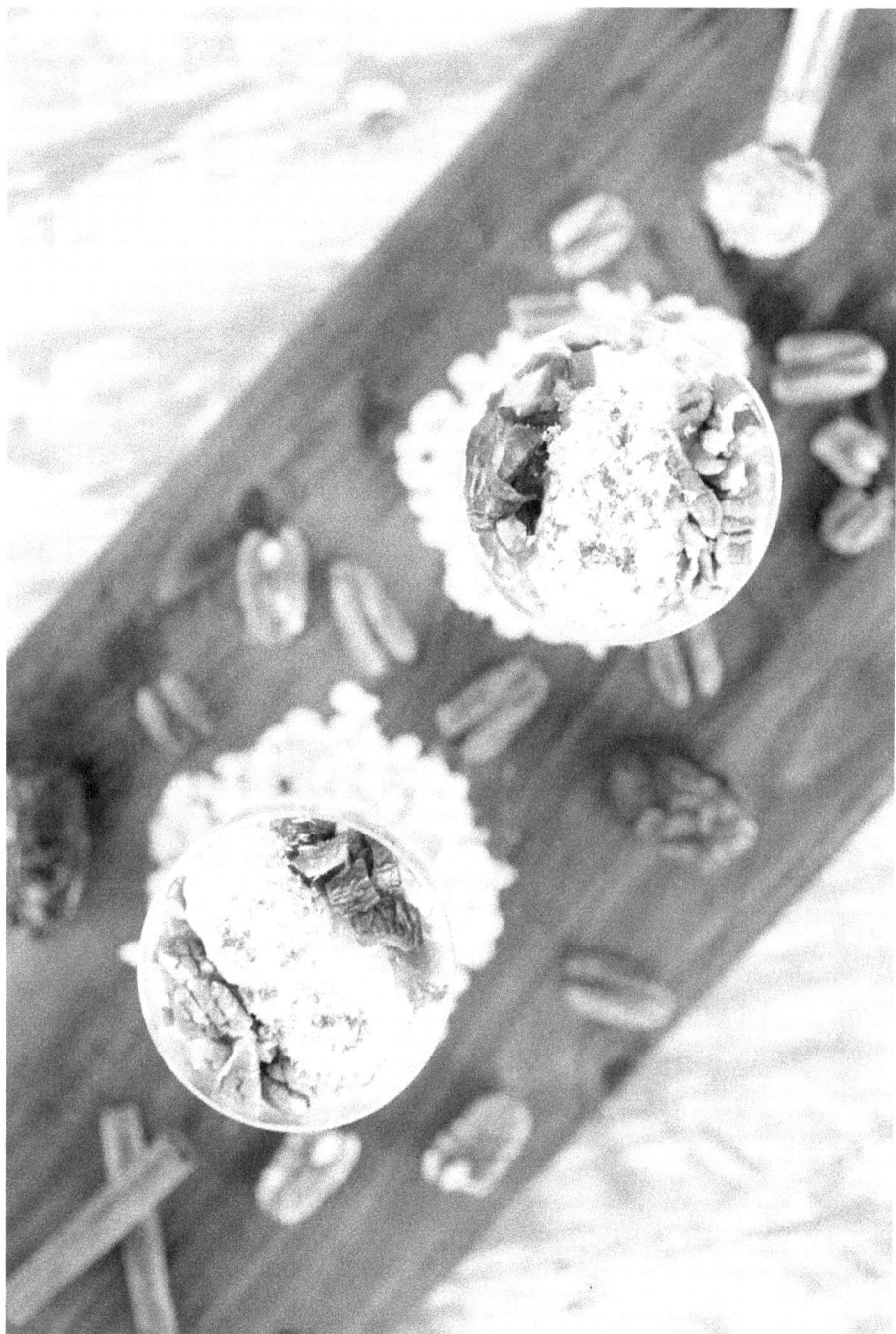

Ingredients

- Oats

- Half of cup unsweetened plain almond milk (or sub other dairy-free milk, such as coconut, soy, or hemp!)
- 3/4 Tbsp of chia seed

- 2 Tbsp of natural salted peanut butter or almond butter (creamy or crunchy // or sub other nut or seed butter)

- 1 Tbsp of maple syrup (or sub coconut sugar, natural brown sugar, or stevia to taste) half of cup gluten-loose rolled oats (rolled oats are best, vs. Steel-cut or quick-cooking) Toppings optional

- Sliced banana, strawberries, or raspberries Flaxseed meal or additional chia seed Granola

Instructions

1.   Take alittle bowl with a lid, add almond milk, chia seeds, spread , and syrup (or every othersweetener) and stir with a spoon to mix . The spread doesn't got to be alright blended with the almond milk (doing so leaves swirls of spread to enjoy the next day).

2.   Add oats and stir a couple of extra times. Then depress with a spoon to form sure all oats were moistened and areimmersed in almond milk.

3.　　Cover tightly with a lid or seal and set within the fridge overnight (or for a minimum of 6 hours) to place/soak.

4.　　the next day, open and knowledge as is or garnish with preferred toppings.
5.　　Overnight oats will preserve within the refrigerator for 2-three days, though high-quality within the primary 12-24 hours in our experience. Not freezer friendly.

Nutrition

Calories: 452, Fat: 22.8g, Saturatedfat: 4.1g, Sodium: 229mgPotassium:

479mgCarbohydrates: 51.7g Fiber: 8.3gSugar: 15.8g Protein: 14.6g

Wedge Salad Skewers

Ingredients

- One head of iceberg lettuce (cut into wedge pieces)

- Four Roma tomatoes cut in half

- One red onion (cut into 1-inch pieces)

- Two avocados cut into 1-inch pieces

- Five slices of bacon cooked and cut into thirds

- One cucumber (sliced (peeled or unpeeled))

- Eight wooden skewers

- Two green onions (diced)

- 1 5 oz container blue cheese crumbles

- One bottle blue cheese dressing

Instructions

1.   One skewer at a time adds an iceberg wedge, tomato, onion, avocado, two pieces of bacon, every other iceberg wedge, and then cucumber.

2.   Continue till all skewers have been made, then garnish with crumbled blue cheese, blue cheese dressing, and diced leafy green onions.

Nutrition

Calories: 238kcal, Fat: 19g, Saturated fat: 6gCholesterol: 25mg Sodium:

401mgPotassium: 573mgCarbohydrates: 10gFiber: 5g Sugar: 3gProtein:

8gVitamin A: 890%Vitamin C: 13.9%Calcium: 144%Iron: 0.9%

Low Sodium Sheet Pan Chicken Fajitas

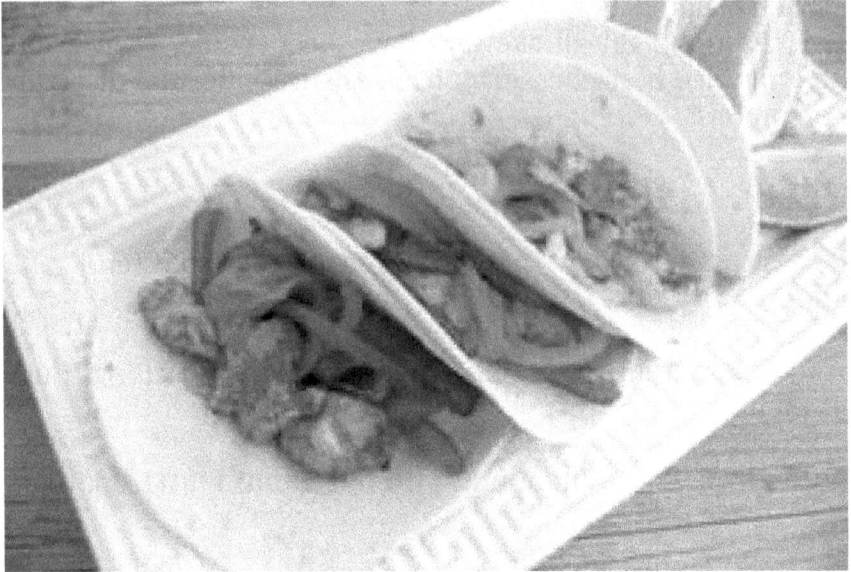

Ingredients

- Two lbs chicken breast tenderloin each sliced in half lengthwise

- One green pepper sliced

- One red bell pepper sliced

- One Vidalia onion sliced

- Olive oil spray

- One tablespoon olive oil Seasoning:

- One teaspoon chili powder

- 1/2 teaspoon smoked paprika

- 1/2 teaspoon garlic powder 1/2 teaspoon onion powder 1/2

- teaspoon dried oregano
- 1/2 teaspoon dried cilantro

- 1/2 teaspoon cumin

- 1/4 teaspoon cayenne pepper

Instructions

1. Preheat oven to 350 degrees F.

2. Apply a coat on a sheet pan with vegetable oil spray.
3. Spread pepper and onion slices onto a prepared sheet pan.
4. Place chicken slices on top of vegetables.
5. Combine seasoning ingredients and stir to mix .
6. Drizzle seasoning mixture over chicken, peppers, and onion.
7. Sprinkle 1 tbsp of vegetable oil over chicken, peppers, and onion.

8.   Gently toss ingredients to distribute seasoning and oil evenly. (make sure chicken strips aren't overlapping)
9.   Bake for 20 min or until chicken reaches 165 deg F.
10.   Serve in warm low sodium tortillas.
11.   Top together with your favorite toppings! i really like cheddar and soured cream .

Nutrition Facts

Calories 168Calories from Fat 36 Fat 4g6% Sodium 140mg6% Potassium 531mg15% Carbohydrates 5g2% Fiber 1g4% Sugar 3g3% Protein 24g48%

Vitamin C 34.3mg42% Calcium 17mg2% Iron 0.8mg4%

Pineapple Protein Smoothie

Ingredients

- 3/4 cup milk

- 3/4 cup pineapple chunks

- 1/2 cup ice

- 3/4 cup canned chickpeas (rinsed and drained)

- 2 tbsp almond butter

- Two pitted dates

- 2 tsp ground turmeric

Directions

Blend all ingredients until smooth.

Nutrients Calories: 461

Spinach Sunshine Smoothie Bowl

Ingredients

- One packed cup baby spinach

- One banana

- 1 cup of orange juice

- 1/2 avocado

- 1/2 cup ice cubes

- Blueberries (optional)

- Diced pineapple (optional)

- Ground flaxseeds (optional)

Directions

Process the spinach, banana, fruit juice , avocado, and ice during a blender until very smooth.

Serve topped with blueberries, diced pineapple, and ground flaxseeds.

Almond Butter Berry Smoothie

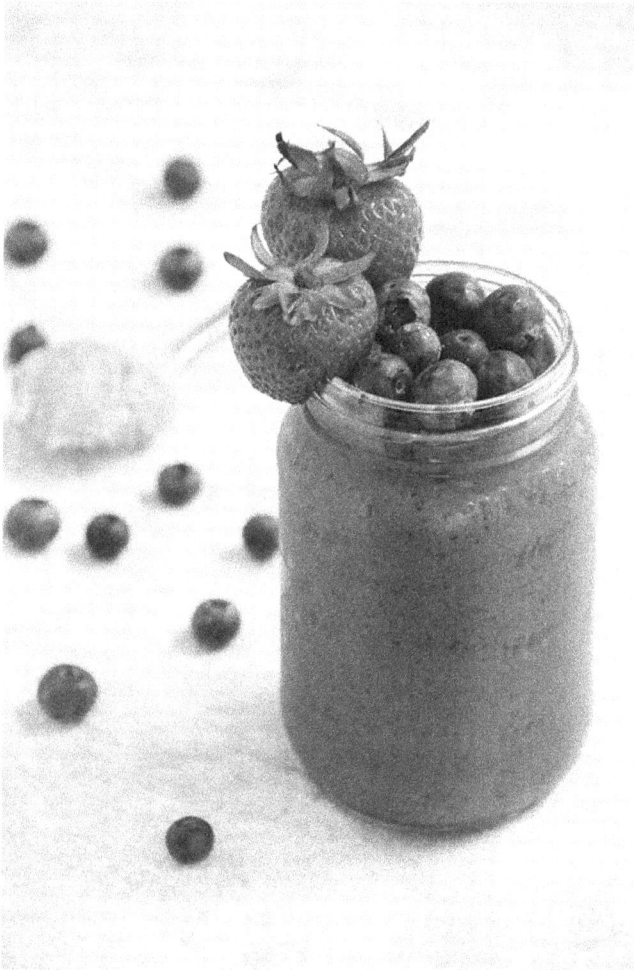

Ingredients

- 1/4 cup 1% low-fat milk

- 1/2 medium ripe banana

- 1 tbsp creamy almond butter

- 1 cup fresh or frozen raspberries

- 1/2 cup crushed ice

Directions

Blend all ingredients until smooth and enjoy!

Pomegranate and Peaches Avocado Toast

Ingredients

- one slice whole-grain bread

- 1/2 avocado

- 1 tbsp ricotta

- Pomegranate seeds, a small amount like one handful Drizzle honey

Directions

1.   Toast the entire grain bread within the oven or toaster.

2.   Spread avocado onto the toast, as smooth or coarse as you favor .

3.   Spread a dollop of ricotta across the avocado.
4.   Drizzle a piece of honey over the avocado mixture.
5.   Sprinkle pomegranate seeds on top and luxuriate in .

Breakfast in a Jar

Ingredients

- 1/4 cup of oatmeal

- 3/4 cup of kefir

- 1 tbsp of chia seeds

- 2 tbsp of raisins

- 1 tbsp of unsweetened coconut flakes

Instructions

Make Layers of elements during a 16-ounce Mason jar , close the lid and

refrigerate overnight.

When it's able to eat, remove the jar from the fridge and provides it a fast stir.

Avocado Egg Cups

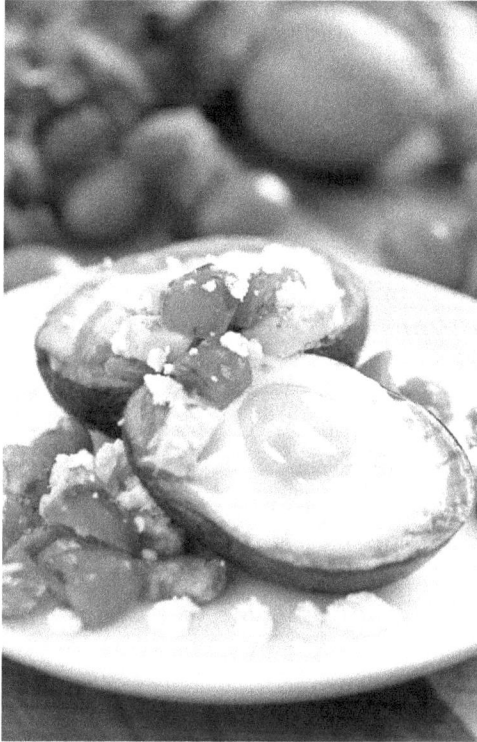

Ingredients

- Two avocados, ripe

- 1/4 tsp coarse salt

- 1/4 tsp pepper

- 1/2 tsp olive oil

- Four medium eggs

1 tbsp grated cheese, such as Parmesan, cheddar, or Swiss
Assorted toppings: herbs, scallions, salsa, diced tomato, crumbled bacon, Sriracha, paprika, crumbled feta

Directions

1.   Heat oven to 375°F. Halve avocados lengthwise and pit. Cut a thin slice from bottom of every avocado half so that it sits level. Where Hell was, scoop out only enough of the flesh (about ½ tbsp) to form room for an egg.

2.   Place avocados on a foil-lined rimmed baking sheet. Season each with salt and pepper, and rub with vegetable oil .

3.   Crack an egg into each cavity (some of the albumen will run over the side, but don't be concerned about it). Sprinkle with cheese, if using. Cover loosely with foil.

4.   Bake almost 20 to 25 min, or until eggs are set to your liking. Sprinkle with toppings.

Sugar Break Apple and Peanut Butter Oatmeal

Ingredients

- 1 cup steel-cut oats

- Three medium-large Granny Smith apples, cored and sliced into 1-2" chunks

- A swirl of peanut butter

- pinch ground cinnamon

- 1 tbsp butter (optional)

- 4 cups of water

- pinch salt

Directions

Cook the oats till they reach the specified texture and creaminess.

Cut apples, toss them into the oats, and stir.

Then add spread into it and stir until melted and spread throughout.

Top with a touch of cinnamon and butter (optional) and enjoy!

Nutrient Calories: 453

Sweet Potato Toast

ù

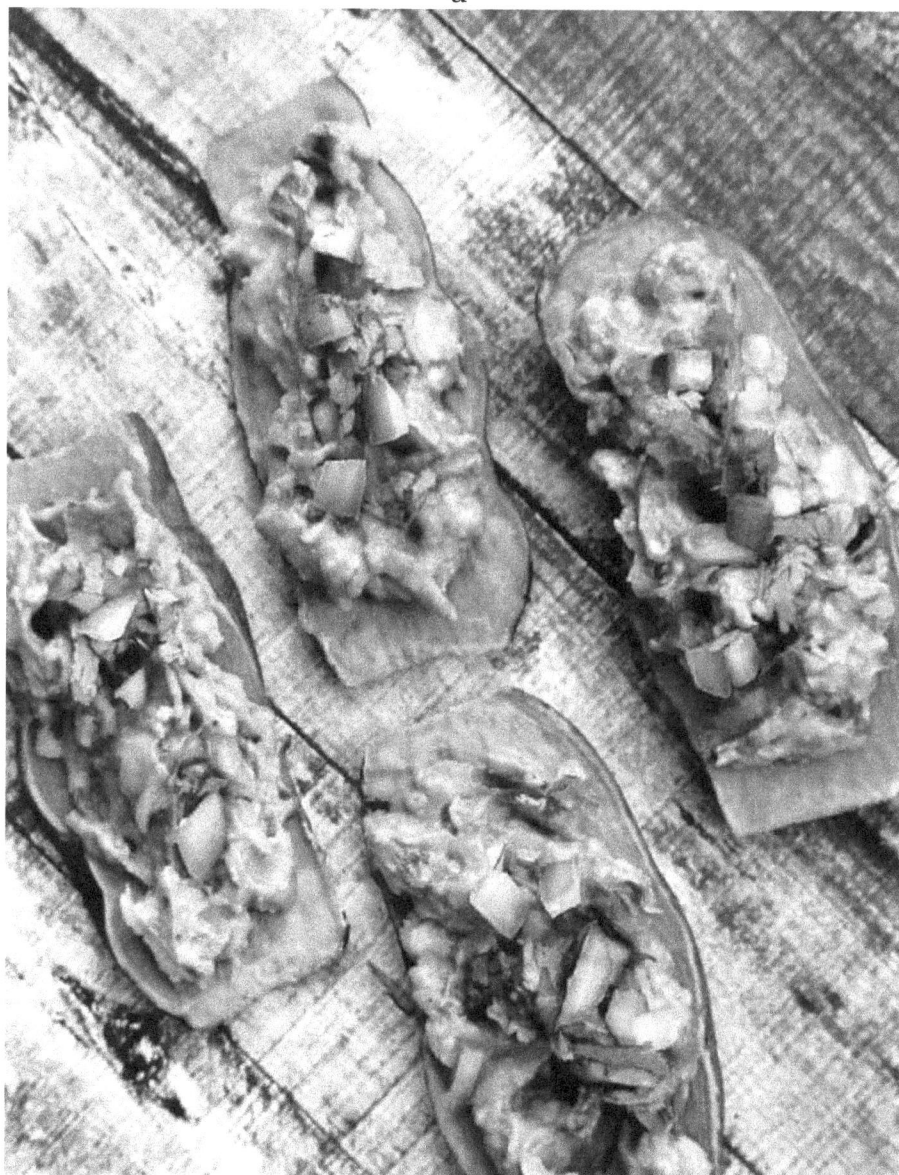

Ingredients

- One potato (sweet)

Instructions

1.   Divide the sweet potato into 1/4-inch slices and pop into the toaster.

2.   Top with anything you select . Popular combinations include spread with fruit, avocado, hummus, eggs,cheese, and tuna fish salad .

Nutrient Calories: 112

Ulli'sGranelli

Ingredients

- 4 cups rolled oats

- 2 cups raw cashews

- 2 cups raw walnuts

- 2 cups of raw almonds

- 2 cups of fresh sunflower seed

- 2 cups of raw pumpkin seeds

- 3 cups unsweetened coconut flakes

- 1/2 cup of maple liquid syrup

- 1/4 cup of unrefined coconut oil, plus

- 2 tsp for oiling the baking sheet

- pinch of sea salt

- 1/3 cup of pure orange oil

- 2 cups of organic raisins

- 2 cups of dried cherries or cranberries

Directions

1.   Set the oven to 300°F.

2.   during a considerable bowl, mix the oats, nuts, seeds, and coconut flakes.

3.   Take alittle bowl, stir together the syrup , copra oil , salt, and orange oil till well combined, then pourover the oat-nut combination and blend nicely.

4.   Spread granola on an outsized oiled baking sheet (do it in batches if needed) and bake for 35-forty minutes untilgolden brown (rotate the baking sheet halfway via for even baking).

5.   Remove from oven and permit refreshing absolutely before mixing with raisins and dried cherries or cranberries.

6.   Store in airtight place within the fridge to stay extra crispiness.

Tofu Turmeric Scramble

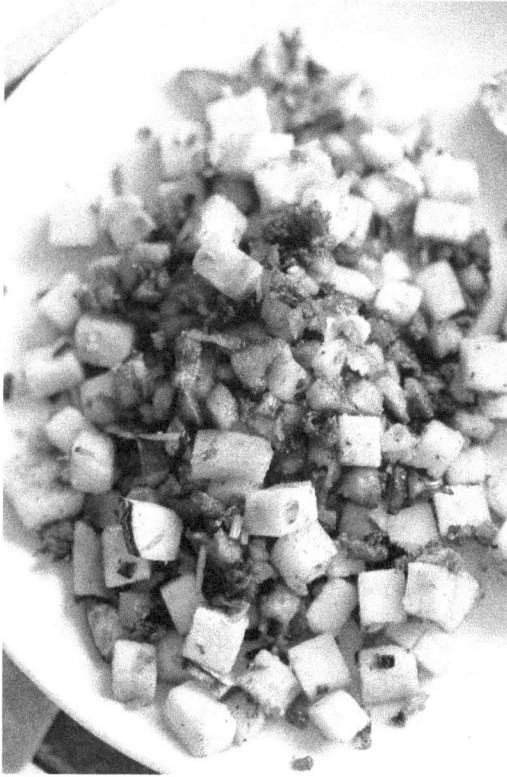

Ingredients

- One 8-ounce block of firm or extra-firm tofu, drained 1 tbsp extra virgin olive oil ¼ red onion, chopped

- One green or purple bell pepper, chopped 2 cups of clean spinach, loosely chopped ½ cup sliced button mushrooms ½ tsp every salt and pepper

- 1 tsp garlic powder

- ½ tbsp turmeric

- ¼ cup nutritional yeast

Directions

1.   Drain the tofu and squeeze lightly to try to to away with extra water. Crumble tofu right into a bowl with the help of hand - the smaller the pieces, the higher .

2.   Prep vegetables and region an outsized skillet at medium temperature. Once ready, then add vegetable oil , onions, and bellpeppers. Mix during a pinch of the salt and pepper and prepare dinner for about five minutes to melt the vegetables. Then add mushrooms and sauté for two mins. Then upload tofu. Sauté for about three minutes, a touch more if the tofu is watery.

3.   Add the remainder of the salt, pepper, garlic turmeric, and nutritional yeast and blend with a spatula, ensuring the spicescombo well. Cook for an additional 5 to eight mins till tofu is lightly browned.

4.   Add the spinach and canopy the pan so as to steam for 2 minutes. Serve immediately with facets of yourchoice.

5.   Nutrient CALORIES: 158

Whole Grain Cheese Pancakes

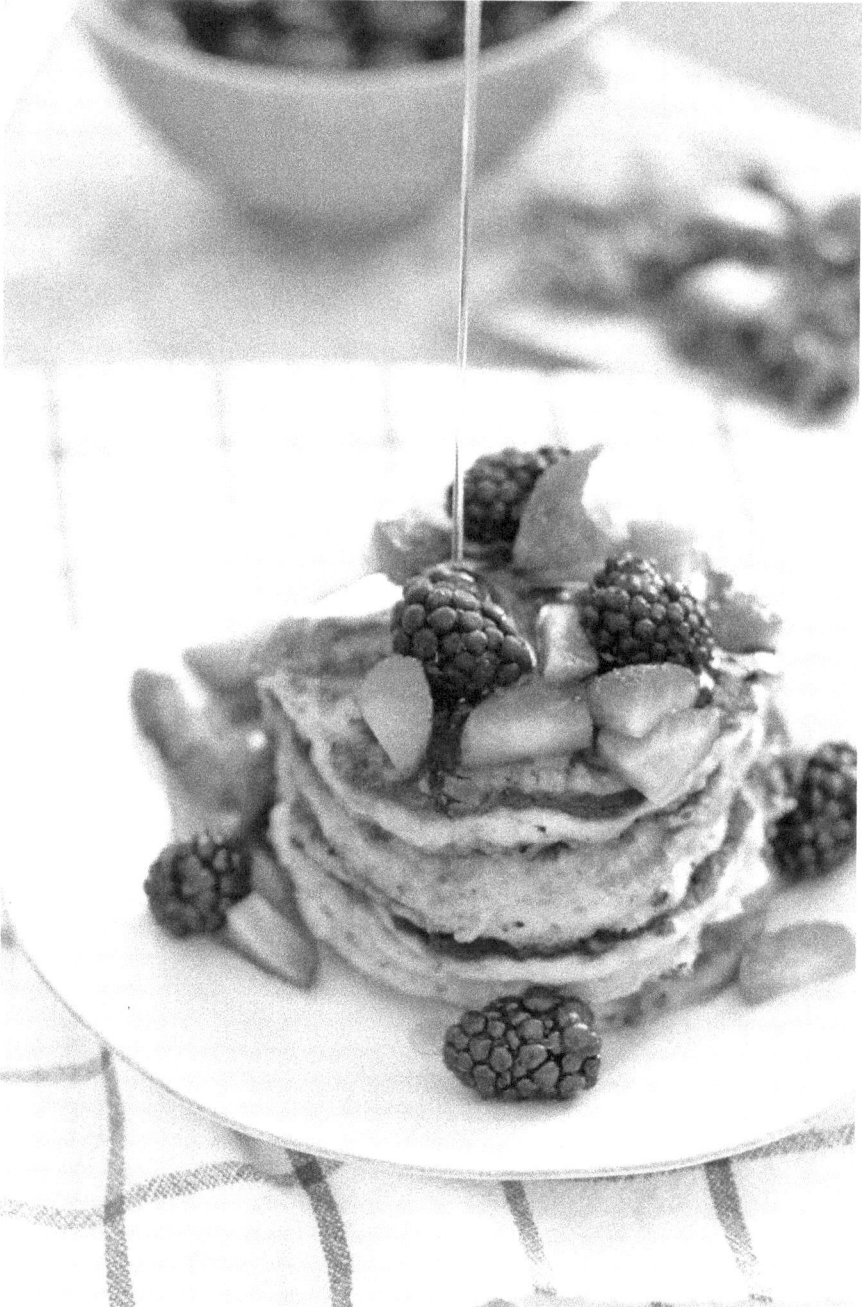

Ingredients

- 1 cup of oat flour

- 1/2 cup of sorghum flour

- 2 tbsp of teff flour

- 1/3 cup of plus 1 tbsp, tapioca starch

- 1 tbsp of baking powder

- 1/2 of tsp salt

- 3 1/2 of tsp sugar

- 1/2 tsp of flax meal

- 3/4 cup of buttermilk

- 1/3 cup of cottage cheese

- Three eggs

- half tsp vanilla extract

- 4 tsp canola oil

- 1-pint blueberries

- 1/2 cup maple syrup

- 3 tbsp water

- 1 tsp lemon juice

- pinch of salt

Instructions

1.   Combine all of your dry elements during a huge bowl and stir to combine evenly.

2.   Whisk all of your wet ingredients in another bowl collectively.
3.   Make a hole within the center of your dry substances and start to slowly pour within the wet materials, a few quartercup at a time. this may confirm that no lumps form when whisking.

4. Continue including your wet components to the flour base till a smooth batter forms. Let the batter relax for quarter-hour at an equivalent time as you preheat your grill.

5. While the grill is warming up, make a warm maple blueberry compote. Mix blueberries, syrup , water,lemon juice, and a pinch salt during a small pot. Stir frivolously to combine .

6. Gently heat the pot over medium-low warmth till the blueberries start to pop and release their natural juices. Setaside, but maintain heat.

7. Once the grill is preheated to a medium-hot temperature, lightly oil the restaurant employing a nonstick spray or asmall amount of neutral-flavored oil.

8. Ladle the batter on to the skillet, ensuring you are doing not overload it.

9. Give time to the pancakes to cook undisturbed until the looks of the sides dry and bubbles come to thesurface without breaking. This has got to take roughly minutes.

10. Flip the pancakes over and cook at the opposite facet for an additional two minutes.

11. Keep heat or serve immediately with the sweet and comfy maple-blueberry compote.

Nutrient Calories: 511

Red Pepper, Kale, and Cheddar Frittata

Ingredients

- 1 tsp olive oil

- 5 oz baby kale and spinach

- One red pepper, diced

- 1/3 cup sliced scallions

- 12 eggs

- 3/4 cup milk

- 1 cup sharp shredded cheddar cheese

- 1/4 tsp salt

- 1/4 tsp pepper

Directions

1. Preheat oven to 375 °F .

2.   Spray an eight 1/2-inch by using 12-inch glass or casserole dish with vegetable oil or nonstick spray.

3.   Heat oil during a large frypan . Add crimson peppers on low and cook until tender. Add kale and spinach, onoccasion stirring till vegetables are wilted, or for about three min.

4.   Transfer peppers and greens to the plate, spreading evenly. Add sliced scallions.

5.   Beat eggs with milk, salt, and pepper. Pour the egg aggregate over the pan. Sprinkle cheese on top.

6.   Bake about 35-40 mins or till the mixture is totally set and starting to lightly brown. For extra color, place under broiler for an extra 1 to 3 minutes, watching to make sure the highest doesn't burn. Let cool about five mins before cutting it.

7.   Serve it as warm or refrigerate for a fast breakfast during the week

— microwave for 1-2 minutes to reheat.

Nutrient CALORIES: 77

Scrambled Eggs with Bell Pepper and Feta

Ingredients

- Olive oil-Salad or cooking-1 tsp-4.5 grams

- Green bell pepper-Sweet, green, raw-2 medium (approx 2-3/4"

- long, 2-1/2" dia)-238 grams
- Egg-Whole, fresh eggs-Four large-200 grams
- Feta cheese-1 oz-28.4 grams

Directions

1.   Heat the oil during a skillet on medium heat. Add chopped peppers and cook till tender.

2.   Stir the eggs and increase the skillet with the peppers. Stir slowly over medium-low heat till they attain your preferred doneness. Sprinkle inside the feta cheese and stir to combine and soften the cheese. Serve directly and luxuriate in it!

Nutrient

Calories 448 Carbs 14g Fat 30g Protein 31g Fiber 4g Net carbs 10g Sodium 551mg Cholesterol 769mg

Devilled Egg Toast

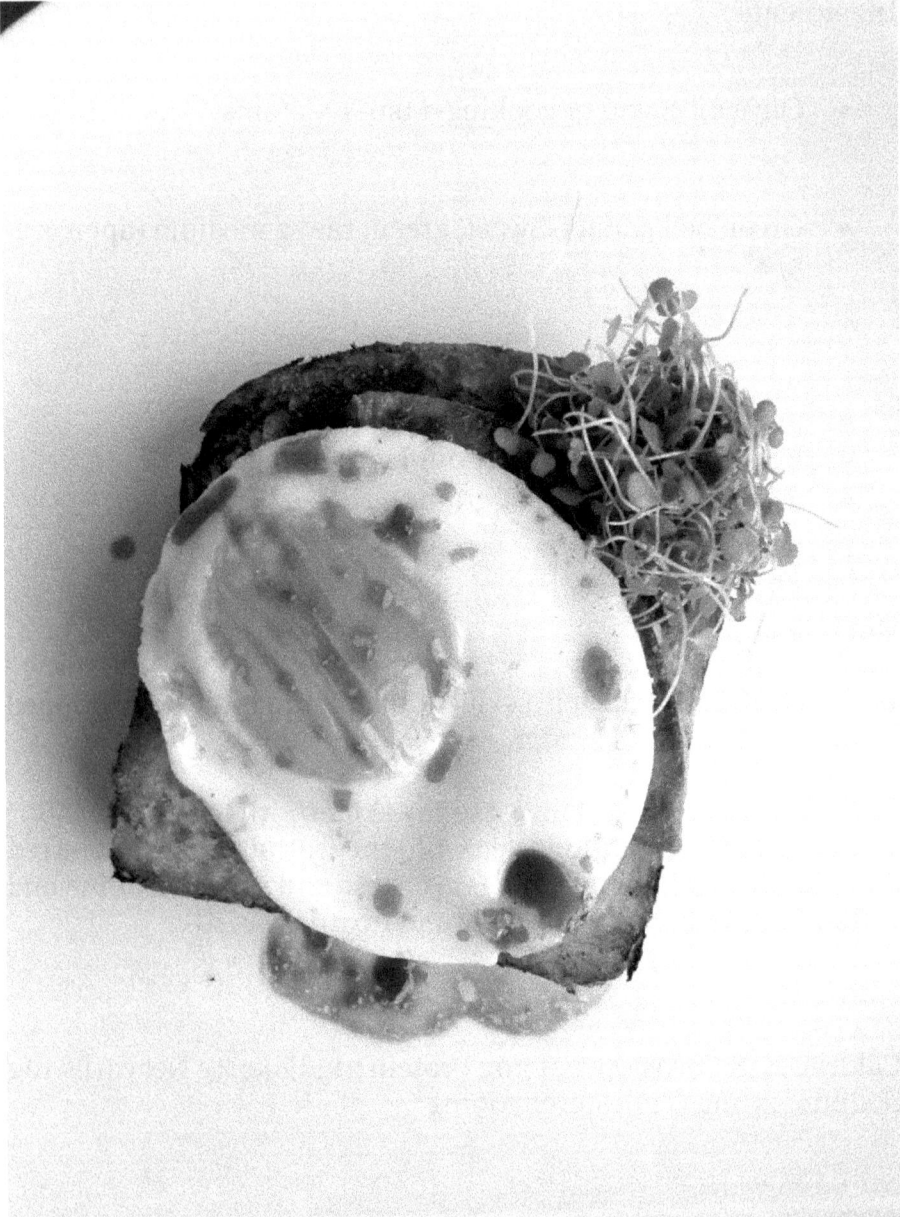

Ingredients

- Egg-Whole, fresh eggs-Two large-100 grams
- Mustard-Prepared, yellow-2 tbsp-30 grams

- Light mayonnaise-Salad dressing, Kraft brand-2 tbsp-30 grams Whole-wheat bread-Commercially prepared-Four slice-112 grams

Directions

1.   Place egg during a bowl and canopy with water. Boil the water, remove from heat, cover, and let sit 10 minutes. Drain under cold water, peel, and mash.
2.   Combine egg with the mustard and mayonnaise. Mix well.
3.   Toast bread and top with egg mixture. Enjoy!

Nutrition

Calories 543 Carbs 53g Fat 24g Protein 28g Fiber 8g Net carbs 45g Sodium 1173mg Cholesterol 382mg

Basic scrambled eggs

Ingredients

- Egg-Whole, fresh eggs-Six large-300 grams

- Butter-Unsalted-1 tbsp-14.2 grams

- Chives-Raw-1 tbsp chopped-3 grams

- Tarragon-Spices, dried-1 tbsp, ground-4.8 grams

- Table-One dash-0.40 grams

- Pepper-Spices, black-One dash-0.10 grams

Directions

1.   Beat the eggs during a bowl and till damaged up. Sprinkle with a pinch each of salt and pepper and beat to include .Place tablespoons of the eggs during a small bowl; put aside .

2.   Heat a 10-inch nonstick frypan over medium-low warmth until hot, approximately 2 minutes. Add butter to the pan and therefore the usage of a rubber spatula, swirl until it's melted and foamy, and therefore the box is flippantly coated. Pour within the massive a part of the eggs, sprinkle with chives and tarragon (if the usage of), and let sit down undisturbed till eggs just start to line round the edges, about 1 to 2 minutes. Using the rubber spatula, push the eggs from the edges into the center . After30

seconds repeat pushing the eggs from the sides into the middle every 30 seconds till simply set, for a complete cooking time of about 5 minutes.

3.   Add the last word tablespoons raw egg and stir till eggs not look wet. Remove from warmness and season with salt and pepper as required . Serve immediately.

Nutrition

Calories 546 Carbs 5g Fat 40g Protein 39g Fiber 0g Net carbs 4g Sodium 586mg Cholesterol 1147mg

Baked Butternut-Squash Rigatoni

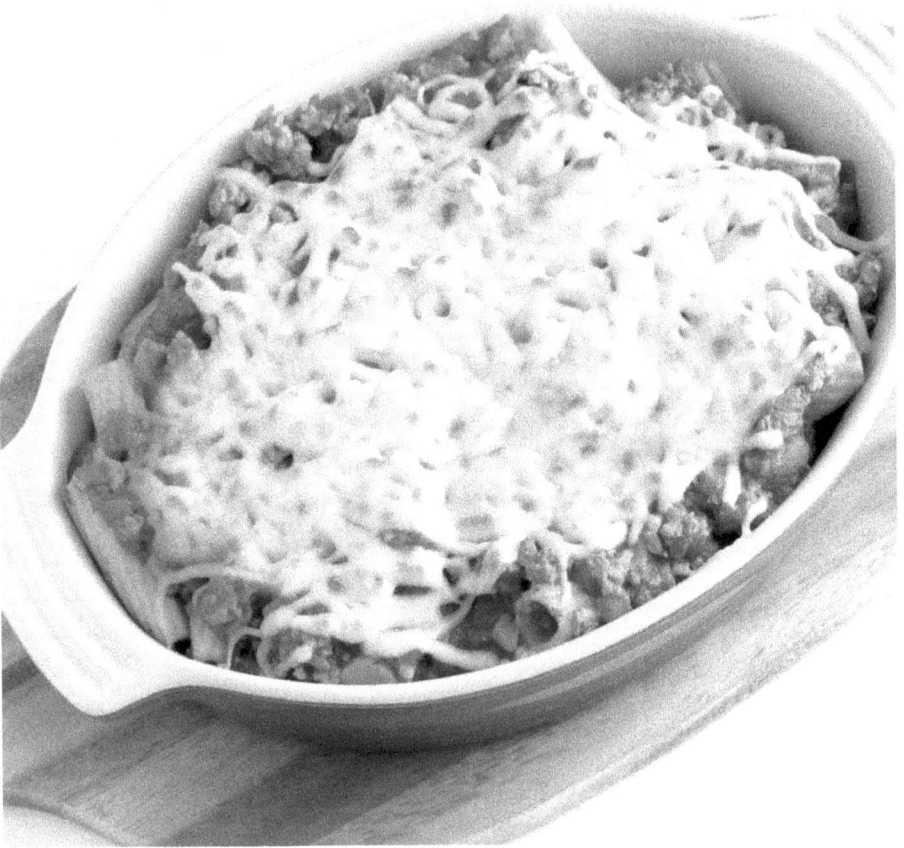

Ingredients

- One large butternut squash

- Three clove garlic

- 2 tbsp. olive oil

- 1 lb. rigatoni

- 1/2 c. heavy cream

- 3 c. shredded fontina

- 2 tbsp. chopped fresh sage

- 1 tbsp. salt

- 1 tsp. freshly ground pepper

- 1 c. panko breadcrumbs

Directions

1.   Set oven at 425 degrees. At an equivalent time, take an outsized bowl and toss garlic, squash, and vegetable oil for coating. Take a baking sheet and roast for about hour . Then calm for 20 minutes. Reduce oven to 350 degrees.

2.   Then, boil the salted water and cook rigatoni consistent with package directions. Drain and put aside .
3.   employing a blender, purée reserved squash with cream until smooth.
4.   Take an outsized bowl and blend squash puree with reserved rigatoni, 2 cups fontina, sage, salt, and pepper. Apply olive oil on the edges of the baking pan. Transfer rigatoni-squash mixture to plate.

5.   Take a little bowl, combine the remaining fontina and panko. Sprinkle over pasta and bake until golden brown,20 to 25 minutes.

www.ingramcontent.com/pod-product-compliance
Lightning Source LLC
Chambersburg PA
CBHW050744030426
42336CB00012B/1653